TUMMY TUCK

ARE YOU THE RIGHT CANDIDATE FOR A TUMMY TUCK

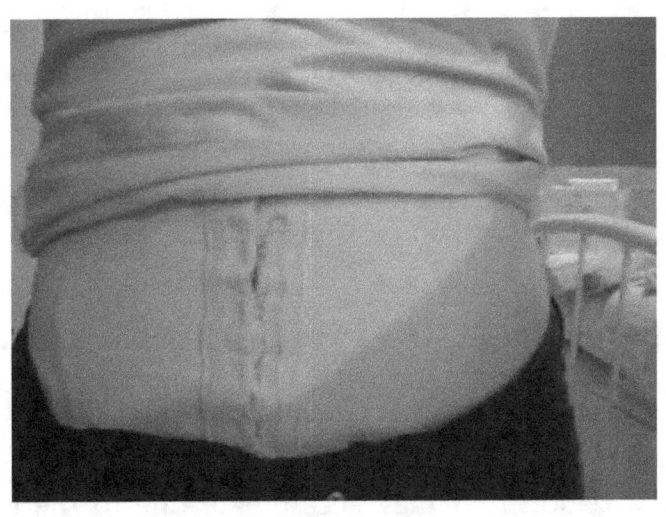

BY TONY WILLIAM

Introduction

I want to thank you and congratulate you for choosing the book, *" TUMMY TUCK: ARE YOU THE RIGHT CANDIDATE FOR A TUMMY TUCK "*.

If you've tried every sit-up and stomach crunching move there is, and are still far from your goal of a flat-as-a-board belly or six pack, then a tummy tuck could be the right choice for you. A tummy tuck, also known as abodominoplasty, is a cosmetic surgery procedure aimed at removing excess flab from the abdominal area, and tightening the abdominal muscles. Like all cosmetic procedures, it's not a "one size fits all" option.

A tummy tuck is not a weight loss measure, and should never be treated like one. It's a procedure for people who want to firm and tone up their abdominal muscles, and have exhausted all their options. A tummy tuck is an invasive surgery, and those who elect to have it should take the time to educate themselves before making a final decision.

A tummy tuck, also known as abdominoplasty, is a cosmetic surgery designed to remove excess skin and fat from the abdominal region that may accumulate due to the effects of pregnancy, obesity, or age. A tummy tuck also restores stretches or weakened abdominal muscles. Tummy tuck operations have been increasing in popularity.

Thanks again for choosing this book, I hope you enjoy it!

ABOUT THE AUTHOR

Mr. Tony William is a Sociologist. He is the CEO of C.E.F Associates and formerly served as head of department of sociology in Premier Natural Resources Inc.

A graduate of University of Toronto with a B.A in Health and Wellness and holds an M.S. from Cambridge University in Health and Fitness and PhD in Social Science.

He has written many articles on health and fitness in different newspapers. He has appeared in many magazines and is frequently interview on skin and body care. He has worked on the importance of health of relationship between parents and children.

He has written other books that focuses on health and wellness of children and what to expect from them at any age level. This book has helped parents understand their children.

C.E.F Associates formed in 1999, has worked both nationally and internationally. This is a consulting company which has clients all over the world. Mr. William is the CEO of the company, and because of his servings in foreign countries the company has a huge client base.

TABLE OF CONTENT

Chapter 1

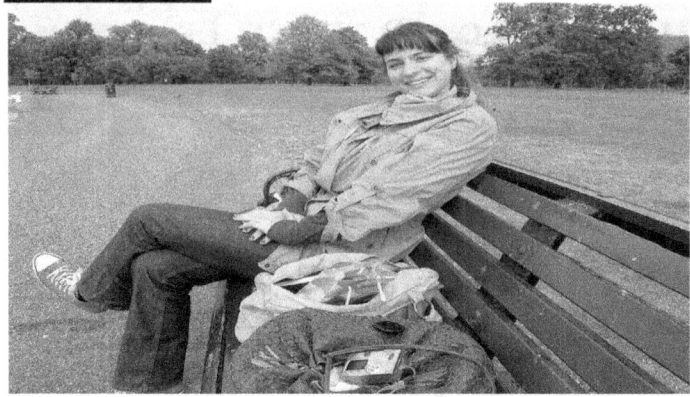

KEY FACTS ABOUT TUMMY TUCKS

You have discovered that ending your relationship with your love handles is harder than finding help in a box store. Your efforts at diet and exercise have not gotten rid of stubborn fatty bulges, and the loose skin from multiple pregnancies or weight loss simply hangs and hangs. For a smoother and shapelier torso your remaining option is the tummy tuck, also know as abdominoplasty.

With a tummy tuck, excess skin and fat are removed surgically from the abdominal region, and the underlying muscles are tightened to create a slimmer and smoother contour. The procedure also better defines the waist. This plastic surgery procedure is a major surgery, and does re□uire some recovery time. Like any plastic surgery, not everyone is a candidate, but if you are considering a tummy tuck, consider these facts about this common cosmetic procedure.

1. Your physical condition determines whether you are a suitable candidate for a tummy tuck. Ideally, men or women who are in reasonably good physical condition make the best candidates for the removal of excess fat bulges and loose skin, especially if they have already tried to get rid of it with diet and exercise.

2. If your excess skin and fat is mostly concentrated below the belly button, you may be a candidate for a mini tummy tuck. In this procedure, there is a shorter incision, and the belly button is not moved. There is also a shorter recovery from a mini tummy tuck than from a standard or full tummy tuck.

3. Because a tummy tuck is a surgery that requires a long incision, you will be left with a scar. To reduce this negative consequence, we place the scar in the lower abdomen that will typically be covered by underwear and bathing suits. And, with proper healing, the scar often becomes very faint.

4. Smoking interferes with recovering from surgery and increases the risks of complications following a tummy tuck. If you are a smoker, you will have to face quitting smoking two weeks before your surgery and during your recovery. Permanently quitting would certainly be best for many reasons.

5. You should be aware that liposuction may be used in conjunction with your tummy tuck. Indeed, liposuction might be all that is needed to achieve the desired result on your abdomen. Be open to the possibility that you may only need the less invasive procedure of liposuction. When you meet your plastic surgeon, he or she will examine you and help determine the best option.

6. When you visit your plastic surgeon for a consultation about a tummy tuck, be candid about your body-shaping goals. Your surgeon will be evaluating the skin and fat deposits of your body along with your expectations about results.

7. The results of a tummy tuck can be very long lasting if you eat sensibly and stay active. If you overeat and gain weight excessively, then your skin and tissues will be forced to stretch out into new bulges.

Chapter 2

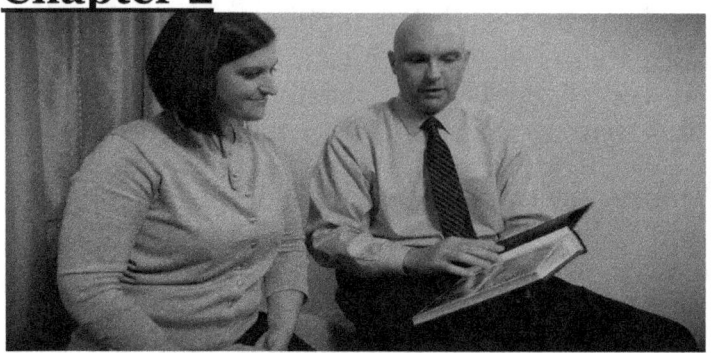

UNDERSTANDING THE TUMMY TUCK PROCEDURE

There are numerous factors which help determine waist size. For some of us, those days of size 2 jeans and bikinis went out the door when we had children. For other, we have struggled all our life to trim our waistline. Time, age, and environmental factors can rob us of the figure we are more comfortable with, and leave us with a very stubborn waistline that won't seem to firm up no matter what we do.

Some of us choose to remedy the situation with what we consider to be a □uick little tummy tuck. Tummy tucks are in fact medical procedures, and while many people are □uite happy with the results, patients who understand the mechanics and expectations after the procedure are more likely to fair much better afterward.

All surgery, including cosmetic surgery, comes with its share of risks. Anesthesia does occasionally throw out a few unexpected complications. However, when we weigh the risks against the benefits, most people feel the risks are small enough to accept. Cosmetic surgery will re□uire ample recovery time.

The recovery times for cosmetic surgery various with each procedure. Obviously a tummy tuck will be more initially restricting than a nose job, although most people can return to work within about two to three weeks. People with more physically demanding jobs may re□uire an extra week or two at home.

The tummy tuck is a medical procedure that re□uires cautious movement in recovery, and ample understanding of the restrictions imposed for recovery prior to going through with this particular cosmetic procedure.

The Tummy Tuck

The tummy tuck is a cosmetic procedure that is based on surgically tightening up the abdominal muscles in order to slim down the waistline. You are essentially "tucking" the unwanted body layers underneath itself much the same way we fold clothes. Naturally it's a little more complicated than that, but you get the idea.

When a cosmetic surgeon begins the tummy tuck process, he/she makes two incisions. One along the hip bone around the pubic area, and the other releases the belly button so it can be reattached in a new position later. The skin is then separated from the torso in order to reveal the muscle underneath. This is where the heart of the tummy tuck occurs. This exposed abdominal muscle is what the surgeon will the stitch into a tighter, reshaped waistline. By tightening up the muscle and actually stitching it in place, new definition to the lower abdomen is formed, and the results are typically a smaller waistline.

The description of the tummy tuck may not sound pleasant, but it is important for patients to understand what is happening to their body so they can recover accordingly. Understanding the procedure prepares patients better, and they often have shorter recovery time because they don't try to take on too much too early.

Recovering from the Tummy Tuck

Recovering from any cosmetic procedure can be a timely process. It is still surgery after all. Tummy tucks take a fair amount of recovery time, and absolutely a time frame that does not allow the patient to lift or carry. The first few days after surgery are the roughest, and the patient must experience the discomfort of the natural bruising and swelling that occurs when the body is rearranged.

Typically it only takes about five day for the incisions to heal after surgery, and the stitches are removed. This does not mean, however, that the patient can then return to anything resembling normal activities. There is still a lot of healing to be done after this type of cosmetic procedure.

The patient will be re□uired to wear a support specifically designed for post tummy tuck recovery time to help the muscles adjust and stay in place, as well as to protect the new waistline from harm while it heals. Most patients report that the support also relieves pain initially as it helps to hold everything in the abdomen in place and relieves stress.

The tummy tuck does leave scars. Most cosmetic procedures will leave minimal scarring, and while the tummy tuck is no different it can take anywhere from nine to twelve months before the scarring has reduced enough to show off the new waistline.

The Benefits of a Tummy Tuck

Tummy tucks are a method of returning a figure, most often, to a pre-child bearing condition. The vast majority of tummy tuck patients are women whose abdomens lost their elasticity due to childbirth. Often the muscles can't regain their original structure which is why simply dieting and exercise may help, but won't work.

We live in a society where overweight and out of shape people often do not receive the same opportunities as healthy looking slender people. For women and men who are trying alternative methods of weight reduction without success, the tummy tuck offers a positive solution.

Just like nose jobs, face lifts, and other cosmetic procedures, tummy tucks are effective tools to bringing about the best physical body possible for any individual wishing to attain a higher level of appearance. There is great debate whether this is an emotionally healthy approach, however a society will not change overnight, and criticism can be fierce.

For the most part tummy tucks are a permanent solution to the battle of the waistline. Although bearing more children may result in terminating the effects of the initial tummy tuck at least partially if not all the way.

With a tummy tuck, you can restore the youthful appearance of your body, as well as get rid of those areas of fatty tissue you are struggling with otherwise. If you are in good physical health and you are a stable weight, you may be a good candidate for this procedure. You should not be a smoker, and have realistic expectations.

Keep in mind that this is not a weight loss tool, though. It will help you to get rid of a few pounds, but that will come in the form of removed skin and fatty tissue. You will need to be in good overall shape to have this procedure done. Your doctors will often re☐uire you to be at a stable weight as well.

Important Considerations

Cosmetic procedures are not for everyone. People who are in very poor physical shape may not recover as ☐uickly or thoroughly as those who exercise regularly. People who are sensitive to anesthesia also may want to seriously consider the risk benefit ratio before having any cosmetic procedure attempted.

Cosmetic surgery is a science and an art. The human body is the canvas and it is important to take into consideration that the canvases are not perfect. Cosmetic surgeons can not guarantee results because our bodies are simply never going to be perfect. Often the cosmetic surgeon can significantly enhance our appearance, but they can not fix everything.

Taking your recovery seriously is one way to help ensure that the expected results become the final results. Whether it's a tummy tuck or a nose job or liposuction, following your surgeon's post operative instructions is imperative to good results.

Prior to attempting the tummy tuck, you should do your very best to get in good shape with strong abdominal muscles. I know we said that we're doing this because exercising wasn't producing the results desired, but at least strengthening your muscles should help not only in shorter recovery periods, but with the over all success of the operation as well.

Talk to your plastic surgeon well in advance about pre-operative exercise that can help him do his job better. Tummy tucks take better on firmer muscles than on loose muscles. Your doctor should be able to advise you of which exercises will target the specific muscles he believes will assist you in your recovery and success.

While you are firming up, remember your diet. Vegetables and protein can help to prepare your body for the cosmetic procedure, but beware of any vegetable containing high amounts of vitamin K in the two weeks prior to your tummy tuck. Vitamin K is a natural blood thinner, and can enhance bleeding during your tummy tuck. Ibuprofen can do this as well.

Preparing your body well for any cosmetic procedure can help your surgeon do a better job and assist your recovery is many ways. After all, you are commencing on the tummy tuck to improve your overall look.

After you have prepared your body, watched your diet, done your exercises, and gone through with the cosmetic procedure it is now time to take special care of yourself. If you can afford it, a few recovery days in a spa or inclusive result can do a world of good toward your final results.

However, perhaps an alternative to an expensive spa if you're lucky, is an especially attentive significant other to tend to your needs during those first few painful days. The rest will do you well and the care can boost your recovery.

Once you have put in the effort throughout your recovery from your tummy tuck, it won't be long before you begin to see actual results. The swelling will reduce and give way to a shapelier you within a couple of short weeks. Over time, your body will heal and slowly reveal its new self.

The scarring will eventually subside and you will be left with a flatter, firmer tummy and a sexier body. After all, that was the point of all this wasn't it? Luckily you will be able to see some results along the way until you are finally recovered from your tummy tuck. If you timed it well, you may even have that brand new shape just as swim suit season comes rolling. Perhaps it's time to hit the beach.

Chapter 3

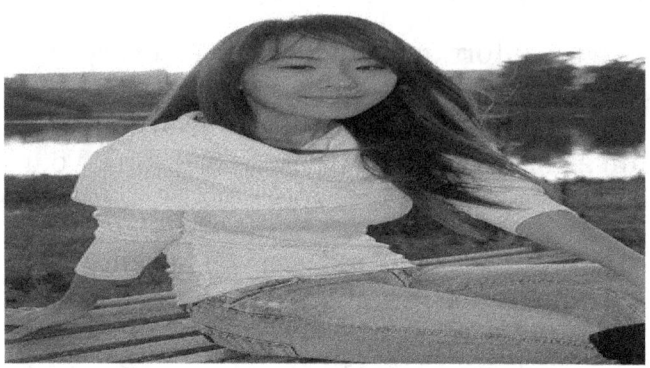

CHOOSING THE RIGHT TUMMY TUCK PROCEDURE

You're standing in front of the mirror, and it seems as though your midsection is glaring back at you. The skin on your stomach is loose, sagging, and you can grab a handful of excess skin. With a frown, you think to yourself where did this come from or how did this happen. Maybe you have lost a significant amount of weight, or maybe your beautiful children wreaked havoc on your midsection during pregnancy. Unfortunately, skin expands, loses tone, and sags as we age, fluctuate in weight, or bear children. Whatever the cause, if you stand in front of the mirror and all you see is your loose midsection then you might be a candidate for a tummy tuck.

Abdominoplasty also known as a tummy tuck is a surgical procedure that focuses on removing the excess skin around the midsection and tightening the underlying abdominal muscles. It is important to understand that a tummy tuck is not meant to help you lose weight as it is not a substitute for a healthy diet and active lifestyle. It's recommended that your weight is consistent for nine to twelve months before undergoing the surgery. Maintaining a healthy weight is essential to long-term results, and failure to do so may negate the results of your procedure. Depending on the type of tummy tuck performed, a combination of excess skin removal, liposuction, and abdominal muscle tightening can be used to give the stomach a flatter, toned, and firmer appearance.

Which type of tummy tuck is right for you?

Ultimately this decision will need to be made in collaboration with your board certified plastic surgeon. The three most popular versions of the tummy tuck include the mini, the traditional, and the extended. Below you will find an overview of the three most common types of tummy tucks performed. Each variation on the tummy tuck will also re□uire different pre-surgery and post-surgery care. The information provided is by no means comprehensive; however, a brief understanding of the three will help you have an active conversation with your board certified plastic surgeon.

The mini tuck

The mini tuck, exactly as its name implies, is used for a minimal amount of skin removal. Typical candidates for a mini tuck are those who have a small amount of excess skin or laxity underneath the belly button. Candidates for a mini tuck are relatively fit and usually are seeking to remove that stubborn pooch of skin that is resistant to diet and exercise. A small incision is made in the pubic region which can easily be hidden by underwear or a bikini. Recovery time is patient-specific; however, most patients can resume normal activity within a week.

A traditional or standard tummy tuck

A traditional or standard tummy tuck is a bit more involved. A traditional tummy tuck is ideal for patients who have a sizeable amount of excess skin above and below the belly button that needs to be removed. Most candidates that fit this profile have typically lost a significant amount of weight, have loose skin, and might have weakened abdominal muscles due to pregnancy. This type of tuck re□uires a larger incision which still should be hidden by underwear or a bikini. Again, recovery times is patient-specific; however, with a traditional tummy tuck allow yourself two to four weeks before resuming normal activities.

Extended OR Expanded Tummy Tuck Surgery

In addition to removing excess fat and skin from the abdominal region, extended or expanded abdominoplasty surgery (also called an expanded abdominoplasty), also removes excess skin and fat from the sides of the waist, hips, and flanks. It is through this surgery that "love handles" can be removed. This type of surgery is best for people who have excess skin and fat not only on their tummies, but also along their sides and back. Due to the extent of the surgery, you should expect a one- or two-night hospital stay and then four weeks' recovery before resuming light activity.

Circumferential Tummy Tuck Surgery

The most dramatic surgery of all abdominoplasty surgeries is the circumferential tummy tuck. This procedure re uires removal of a lot more skin than any other form of abdominoplasty procedure. This type of surgery is best for men and women who have lost a significant amount of weight (100+ pounds), and are left with a great deal of loose, sagging skin all over their body

Endoscopic Tummy Tuck

Sometimes considered a "scarless" abdominoplasty procedure, this procedure is similar to having a mini abdominoplasty, but without the large scar. This type of procedure is performed with the use of a special scope that re uires only a small incision for insertion. This surgery is best for those who have a small amount of tummy bulging, very little sagging skin, and great skin elasticity.

A tummy tuck is a highly individualized surgical procedure that re uires expert consultation. When deciding to have a tummy tuck picking the right board certified plastic surgeon to perform the procedure is crucial. Your specific needs and desired results will determine which type of tummy tuck is right for you. At your consultation, your board certified plastic surgeon will discuss which procedure will be most beneficial to achieve your desired results.

Chapter 4

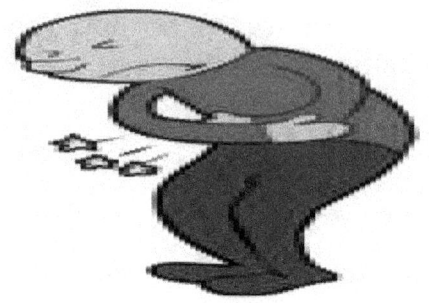

SIX SIGNS YOU'RE A GOOD CANDIDATE FOR A TUMMY TUCK

Like many men and women, you may be dissatisfied with your figure. Despite eating a healthy diet and exercising regularly, you cannot seem to get rid of the excess fat and skin around your belly. Fortunately, a tummy tuck can help you achieve the sleek figure you desire. During this procedure, a cosmetic surgeon will remove excess skin and fat. He or she will also carefully tighten weakened muscles and repair those that have become separated. There are several signs that may indicate your a candidacy for a tummy tuck:

1. You have loose skin around your abdomen

Although a tummy tuck can certainly target stubborn pockets of fat, to □ualify for this procedure, you must also have a significant amount of excess skin around your abdomen. A plastic surgeon will create a fairly sizeable incision to perform a tummy tuck, and if you do not have enough excess skin, it can cause tension in the scar, leading to an unsightly "stretched" look. Both full and partial tummy tucks are available, so if you only have excess skin below your belly button, you may still be a candidate for the latter procedure.

If your skin has little to no elasticity, the only way to improve its appearance is by having a tummy tuck done. The reason why this procedure is needed is because removing fat from behind loose skin won't change the appearance. Therefore, diet and exercise won't make a difference – at least in looks. Skin laxity is caused by a number of factors, including pregnancy and significant weight loss.

If you think that a tummy tuck may benefit your appearance and improve your self-confidence, schedule a consultation with Plastic Surgery Clinic. They are more than happy to discuss the pros and cons to this procedure and if it will help you achieve your long-term goals.

2. You have overall good health

Although tummy tucks are low-risk procedures, you should not undergo this surgery if you have any serious underlying health issues. Because you will be sedated with general anesthesia, you must have a healthy heart and lungs. Additionally, autoimmune disorders and connective tissue disorders can cause serious problems with the healing process. Finally, if your skin typically develops thick, raised scars, you should discuss this with your doctor before undergoing a tummy tuck.

3. You have realistic expectations for the surgery

Although tummy tucks can have a remarkable impact on your appearance and self-confidence, they are not intended to be a weight-loss surgery. You should be aware that following your surgery, you will face a significant amount of recovery time, and your results will appear gradually as your healing progresses. To maintain the results of your tummy tuck, you will need to eat a healthy diet, and maintain a regular exercise routine. If you are committed to a healthy lifestyle, you are likely an excellent candidate for this procedure.

4. You have had a baby or lost a significant amount of weight

Both pregnancy and obesity can cause damage to the abdominal muscles and can stretch the skin around the belly. The skin and muscles are permanently damaged, and even after a patient delivers the baby or reaches a healthy weight range, the tissues will continue to hang loosely around the stomach. A tummy tuck can repair these tissues so that your body will more accurately reflect your healthy weight range.

5. You are not planning on becoming pregnant

If you are planning to have more children, you should wait to undergo a tummy tuck. Future pregnancies can separate the repaired muscles and re-stretch the skin around your belly, meaning you will have to undergo another procedure to restore the results of your first tummy tuck. However, if you do have an unexpected pregnancy, your previous tummy tuck will not affect the health of your baby.

6. You are not planning on losing more weight

You should be within 15 to 20 pounds of your ideal weight before undergoing a tummy tuck. While many patients do lose some weight after the procedure, if you lose more than 30 pounds, it can leave more excess skin and sagging muscles around your stomach, negating the results of your procedure.

7. If your skin has little to no elasticity

The only way to improve its appearance is by having a tummy tuck done. The reason why this procedure is needed is because removing fat from behind loose skin won't change the appearance. Therefore, diet and exercise won't make a difference – at least in looks. Skin laxity is caused by a number of factors, including pregnancy and significant weight loss.

If you think that a tummy tuck may benefit your appearance and improve your self-confidence, schedule a consultation with a Plastic Surgery Clinic. They are more than happy to discuss the pros and cons to this procedure, and if it will help you achieve your long-term goals.

8. You only feel comfortable wearing maternity-style shirts

Maternity shirts are fine in your post-partum days and even while nursing, but if it's all you can wear, you may benefit from a tummy tuck. Not only will this procedure provide you with a firmer, flatter stomach, but also give you confidence. There's no reason why you have to wear maternity clothes long after giving birth.

HOW TO TELL IF YOU'RE THE BEST CANDIDATE FOR A TUMMY TUCK PROCEDURE

When people talk about tummy tuck surgery, you could almost be forgiven for thinking it's some sort of miracle operation that will change you overnight with no obvious after effects. In fact, nothing could be further from the truth. Undergoing a tummy tuck procedure is a major surgical procedure, and a great deal of thought should go into the decision to go ahead.

For starters, are you the best candidate for having a tummy tuck? This isn't some sort of rapid weight loss surgery - in fact, it's mostly suitable for people with an excess of skin in the abdominal region. This has usually been caused by multiple pregnancies or the loss of a great deal of weight. When the abdominal muscles have been repeatedly or extensively stretched, they may struggle to regain their elasticity, leading to sagging skin and an unsightly abdomen. The procedure can also help improve the skin's appearance where the patient has excessive sub-navel stretch marks.

Any candidate for a tummy tuck needs to be in good physical health. It's also important to realize that you will be left with permanent scarring after the operation, and you also have to accept all the usual risks involved in undergoing a general anesthetic. An abdominoplasty re□uires months of recovery time, as well as careful preparation prior to the operation, and good post-operative care.

If you're planning further pregnancies, or intending to lose a significant amount of weight, then a tummy tuck isn't a good idea. You are better off postponing the surgery, or else you risk having the vertical abdominal muscles separate, which re□uires more surgery to repair. If you've already had some type of abdominal surgery, your surgeon may advise against a tummy tuck, or you may find that the new scars are a great deal more visible than you expected.

You also need to think about how a tummy tuck will affect your life in general. Yes, your general state of health needs to be good in order to have the surgery, but you need to allow time to prepare for the operation, as well as being able to take life easy for many months afterwards. This can be particularly difficult if you have dependents, or your job re□uires you to be very active. After the operation you will most likely find yourself physically unable to care for others, and may find your energy levels are substantially lower than normal.

If you have strong abdominal muscles and good health, then your recovery time will be on the shorter end of the scale, but some patients take as many as eight months to get completely back to normal. During this time they may be unable to drive or lift any heavy objects. If you know you can't afford to be restricted for such a long period, then perhaps you should consider waiting to have a tummy tuck until your circumstances will allow you an extended recovery period. Make sure you have discussed the operation with family and friends, as you may find yourself needing their support in the months to come.

Although abdominoplasty can improve the appearance of your abdomen, it's important to realize this isn't a miracle operation. It may help to improve your self-confidence, but you still need to be realistic about the results of the surgery. Make sure you've discussed the operation fully with your surgeon, and also discussed the expected outcomes, so that you're not left believing that a tummy tuck will achieve things that are impossible.

ARE ABDOMINOPLASTY SURGERY AND TUMMY TUCK THE SAME PROCEDURE

There is often times confusion when it comes to the terms abdominoplasty surgery and tummy tuck. Although some people think they are two separate procedures, they really are the exact same procedure. The word abdominoplasty is just a fancy medical term to describe the popular cosmetic procedure that helps patients achieve a flatter stomach. The word tummy tuck is the layman term that is well-known among the general public.

What is the purpose of abdominoplasty surgery?

The purpose of a tummy tuck or abdominoplasty is to remove excess folds of abdominal skin. This helps patients achieve a flatter stomach. The procedure can also help tighten the muscles of the abdomen. This adds to the firmer, flatter appearance of the stomach that patients seek.

Although abdominoplasty can eliminate stretch marks, it cannot get rid of all of them. This is because only the stretch marks located on the fold of skin are able to be removed. All other stretch marks on the abdomen will be left in place, as there is only so much skin that can be removed.

When Abdominoplasty May Be the Only Option

Most patients that undergo abdominoplasty do so because it is the only way to achieve a flat appearance of the stomach. This is because they have excess folds of skin in the abdominal region that diet and exercise cannot eliminate. These loose folds of skin are often the result of one or more of the following:

• Significant weight gain and weight loss

• Multiple pregnancies

• Our genes

• Old age

The purpose of abdominoplasty surgery is not to act as a substitute or alternative for exercise and diet. Patients who wish to undergo abdominoplasty need to be at their ideal weight before undergoing the procedure. Some surgeons will not perform the procedure otherwise. Women who plan on having more children should also postpone the procedure until after they are done having kids. Following these recommendations can help patients achieve the best results possible when then finally do undergo their abdominoplasty surgery.

Is abdominoplasty surgery something you should undergo?

It's important to keep in mind that abdominoplasty is surgery. And like any surgery, it has its risks. This is why you should only undergo the procedure when you feel the benefits of the procedure outweigh the risks involved. Your reason for choosing to undergo abdominoplasty surgery should also be based on what you want-not what someone else wants for you. It's also important to keep in mind that trying to achieve the body of someone you admire is not a good reason to undergo such a procedure. The following are what make a patient a good candidate for the procedure:

* A protruding abdomen which is out of proportion to the rest of your body.

* Loose or sagging abdominal skin.

* Abdominal muscles which are bulging due to age or previous pregnancy.

* Excess body fat located in the abdominal area.

Generally, candidates should not be:

* Overweight

* Smokers

* Women who are or may become pregnant.

A Plastic Surgery Consultation Appointment

If you believe you are a good candidate for a tummy tuck, or if you would like to explore other options such as liposuction, the best thing you can do is to schedule an appointment with a Board Certified plastic surgeon in your local area.

At your consultation appointment the plastic surgeon will go over all of your options after evaluating your body, and listening to your desired results after surgery. You should arrive at your consultation appointment a little early and be prepared to fill out new-patient paperwork.

Once you meet with the plastic surgeon you will be expected to share information on your health history, surgical history, and any, and all medications or supplements you might be taking.

For tummy tuck evaluation appointments you can expect the plastic surgeon to examine your abdomen to check...

- o The □uality of your abdominal skin
- o The elasticity of your abdominal skin.
- o The amount and location of any excess fat and skin.
- o The status of your abdominal wall muscles.
- o And to check for any previous surgical scars.

Once the plastic surgeon has evaluated your physical and emotional health at your consultation appointment, he can then make recommendations to you.

Chapter 5

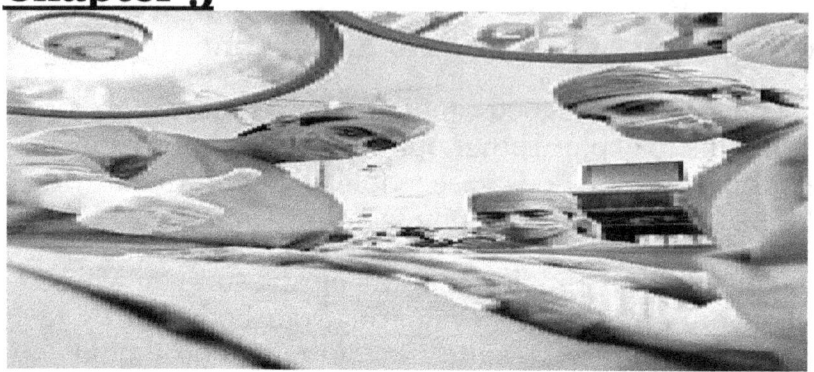

PRECAUTIONS TO TAKE BEFORE AND AFTER THE PROCEDURE

Tummy tuck surgery is the ideal procedure if you are looking to get rid of excess abdominal fat and skin. This cosmetic surgery involves the liposuction process by which surplus fat deposits are effectively removed. Reliable plastic surgery practices utilize advanced devices such as Smartlipo Triplex, BodyTite and VASER 2.0 to perform the procedure and deliver optimal results. However, you have to keep in mind the precautions to take before and after the tummy tuck procedure for the best outcome and safe recovery.

Preparation before the Surgery

Some of the things to be kept in mind before undergoing the tummy tuck surgery include the following:

> ➢ Have a look at the blogs or forums depicting earlier candidate experiences to be confident enough to handle similar situations.
> ➢ Keep your mindset ready for a surgery and seek proper consultation.
> ➢ A drastic diet before the surgery is not recommended.
> ➢ Talk to your surgeon about the medications you usually take and he will guide you on what to take and what not to.

- ➤ It is advisable to ☐uit smoking at least a few weeks before the surgery.
- ➤ Get your home ready with necessary things such as ice packs, petroleum jelly, handheld shower head, loose clothing etc.
- ➤ Arrange for someone to take you home after the surgery as you won't be able to drive alone.
- ➤ Always be realistic about the results of the surgery.

Precautions after the Surgery

After care to enhance the effectiveness of the surgery, and to ensure good results include the following:

- o Follow a balanced diet and take plenty of rest following the surgery for ☐uick healing.

- o It will be good to have more of raw fruits and increase fluid intake.

- o The pain medications taken should be approved by your surgeon.

- o Avoid drinking alcohol and smoking, so as not to hinder the healing process.

- o Lifting materials of an above average weight is not recommended for about 6 weeks.

- o Avoid giving strain to the abdominal muscles via exercise or other activity for 6 weeks. Follow healthy exercise patterns as per the instructions from the surgeon.
- o Resume your normal work in 2-4 weeks, specifically as advised by the surgeon.
- o Exposing your scars to the sun may affect the ☐uick healing process
- o The incisions are to be kept clean to avoid infection that may lead to other complications
- o Antibacterial soaps should be used for body wash to keep incisions clean.

- Avoid giving tension on the incision while sleeping by maintaining the right posture.
- If you don't feel comfortable with the healing process, you may seek necessary instructions from the plastic surgeon .

These are the precautions to be taken before and after the tummy tuck procedure which will not only ensure a safe surgery, but also help you benefit from impressive results. You can achieve a flatter, firmer abdomen with a narrower waistline that will make you look and feel great in your favorite outfits.

Chapter 6

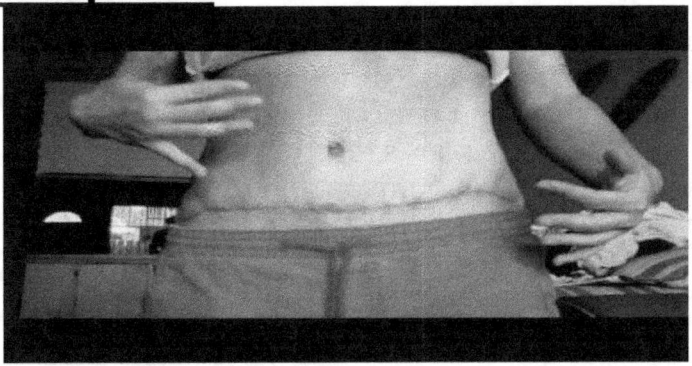

HOW TO REMOVE THE SCARS FROM A TUMMY TUCK

Undergoing a tummy tuck, or abdominoplasty, procedure eliminates excess fat in the abdominal region while tightening your stomach muscles in the process. The surgery involves an invasive incision in your lower abdomen that spans the length of your bikini line, leaving behind an unattractive scar. Although plastic and cosmetic surgeons attempt to minimize scarring, you may not be able to fully remove your tummy tuck scar after your incision has healed. However, some techni☐ues may aid in healing your skin and decreasing the appearance of your scar.

Step 1

Talk to your doctor about surgical scar revision. This method removes the scar by reconnects the unaffected skin, reducing the scars appearance. Surgical scar revision works best for long or wide scars, since the techni☐ue can thin or shorten the scar. Irregular incision lines, rather than a straight incision, is used to make a scar less noticeable. Wait six months to a year after surgery before attempting scar revision.

Step 2

Discuss punch grafts with your physician or surgeon. This procedure involves removing the scar from the skin by cutting a hole around it, explains the American Academy of Dermatology. The site of the scar is then replaced with unscarred skin, generally taken from an unnoticeable spot on the body, such as behind the ear. Healing time is approximately one week as the skin heals. A new scar may form, but the skin is smoother and less visible than deep scars.

Step 3

Undergo laser treatment to remove the scar from your tummy tuck. The laser treatment process involves using a high-energy light to remove or reform skin damaged by a scar. The type of laser depends on the severity and depth of the scar. The procedure is costly, and thick or raised scars need at least two treatments every few months.

Step 4

Give yourself time to recover before focusing on the appearance of your scar. The healing process can take three to six months before the scar flattens or lightens in color, according to the National Institutes of Health.

Tips

Quit or avoid smoking two weeks before your tummy tuck surgery and until the incision heals properly. Smoking puts you at risk of developing complications or infection after the procedure. Complications or infections may slow the healing process and effect the appearance of scarring.

Cover your scar when spending time in the sun. Direct sunlight can cause dark discoloration to your scar while reducing the healing process. Always wear sunscreen or sun block of SPF 15 or higher when you are outside.

Chapter 7

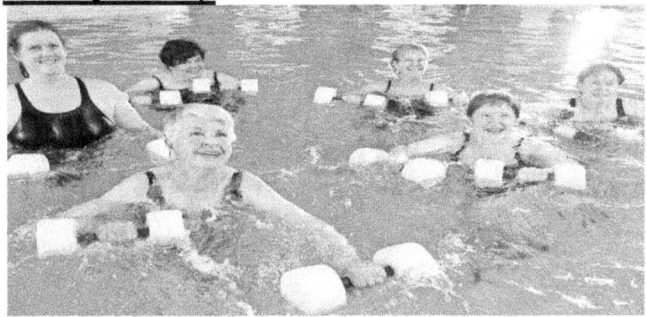

TUMMY TUCK EXERCISES

Would you like a tummy tuck without having to go through surgery? Clinically known as abdominoplasty, tummy tucks remove excess skin and fat and repair muscles in the abdominal wall that may be stretched out from pregnancy, aging, or large fluctuations in weight.

The good news is that many of the results of an actual tummy tuck can be achieved through exercise and diet. And if you've actually had an abdominoplasty, it's important to maintain those results once you've recovered from your surgery.

A pooching stomach is probably a combination of excess weight and underdeveloped abdominal muscles. Exercise can give your abs definition, but if your six-pack is hidden beneath a layer of fat, nobody's going to see it. More importantly, fat around the middle isn't just unsightly, it's unhealthy, with adverse effects on blood pressure, cholesterol, and triglyceride levels and increased risk of diabetes.

There is no such thing as spot reduction – that is, losing weight in a targeted area, and alas, calorie reduction is non-negotiable. You must reduce your calorie intake below what you burn daily to lose fat. Cardio and strength training will help you build and conserve muscle mass while you're losing weight.

Tucking the Tummy

Exercises that require you to tuck your tummy in during the movement are a great place to start for pulling in your waistline. Some of these exercises, such as hollowing and bracing, may seem fairly passive, but do them consistently and it's quite possible their benefits will far exceed the amount of effort they seem to require.

Abdominal Hollowing

Also known as the drawing-in maneuver and stomach vacuum, this exercise is performed by contracting your stomach into your lower spine as far as it can go and holding it. Breathe lightly while holding the pose. Abdominal hollowing can be done sitting, standing or lying down. Hollowing works the transverse abdominus, the deepest-lying of the abdominal muscles, and prevents and reduces back pain.

Abdominal Bracing

Bracing is what you do when you're holding plank position and squeezing your stomach muscles tight. This strengthens the obliques and the rectus abdominus, which is the sheath of muscle where ab definition is most visible.

Also known as crunches, curl-ups work the upper part of the rectus abdominus. Lie face-up on the floor with your knees bent and feet planted hip-distance apart. With your hands behind your head, flex your waist to raise your upper torso from the floor. Keep your lower back on floor or mat and raise torso up as high as possible.

Leg-Lifts

Lie on your back on a floor or bench. With your knees knees straight, lift your legs by flexing your hips until they are extended to the ceiling. Lower your legs until your hips and knees hover just above the surface of the mat or bench. You must bend at your hips to engage the rectus abdominis, the front abdominal muscle.

HOW TO EXERCISE AFTER TUMMY TUCK PROCEDURES

A tummy tuck, medically known as an abdominoplasty, is an invasive surgical procedure performed to remove unwanted fat around the abdomen. The procedure also removes excess skin and aims to tighten abdominal muscles. Consult your physician before attempting an exercise routine after a tummy tuck, as your sutures and muscles need plenty of time to rest and recover from the surgery. The National Institutes of Health recommends avoiding vigorous exercise or heavy lifting for four weeks after a tummy tuck procedure.

Step 1

Sit up on your own and bring yourself to a standing position, several times a day. While this may not seem like a difficult task, it causes your body to work your weakened muscles. Stand with your back straight, as tall as you can, on your own. Ask your caregiver to be present when you first attempt to sit up or get out of bed on your own.

Step 2

Take short walks. Walking or moving around, even for a short amount of time, helps prevent the formation of blood clots. Start walking around your hospital room or house as soon as possible after surgery. As your endurance and strength return, take longer walks around your neighborhood or on a nearby walking path.

Step 3

Start with light cardiovascular exercise four weeks after the procedure. Perform low-impact exercises, such as cycling, using the elliptical and brisk walking.

Step 4

Begin performing upper-body and leg-strengthening exercises around one month after surgery.

Avoid doing exercises that specifically target your abdominal muscles until your muscle strength returns in other areas of the body. This will help you to avoid straining your stomach muscles.

Step 5

Strengthen your abdominal muscles with simple exercises, such as pelvic thrusts and leg slides. As your abdominal strength improves, move on to various types of crunches, planks and leg lifts. Perform one set of 10 to 12 repetitions of each exercise. Add additional sets as strength and stamina increase.

Step 6

Resume your regular exercise program when you've received clearance from your physician. Keep in mind that this may take several months.

Warnings

Give yourself plenty of time to heal after a tummy tuck procedure. Failure to do so may result in severe complications, such as blood loss or clots, infections or scar tissue.

CONSEQUENCES OF WEIGHT GAIN AFTER HAVING A TUMMY TUCK

A tummy tuck, also referred to as abdominoplasty, removes excess skin and then repositions the belly button. It can flatten and firm the abdominal region, but you must also maintain a healthy lifestyle with proper diet and exercise. Minimal weight gain after a tummy tuck will not have a significant impact, but excessive weight gain will stretch the skin and stretch the abdominal muscles. Pregnancy after a tummy tuck can also affect the results.

Stretched Skin

Weight gain after a tummy tuck will affect the surgery results. Since a tummy tuck removes fat cells, there are fewer fat cells in the abdominal area. This means that the fat distribution will be less in the area of the stomach than before, but the skin will stretch and with time there will be more skin.

Loss of Muscle Firmness

Excessive weight gain causes the skin and the abdominal muscles to stretch. This results in a loss of muscle firmness and tone. The abdominals will not remain as flat as they were after the tummy tuck was initially performed.

Regular exercise and a healthy diet are recommended to help maintain the results of the tummy tuck surgery. Abdominoplasty is not a replacement for weight loss. It used to remove excess skin after a large amount of weight loss and/or multiple pregnancies. It can also help people who cannot lose the excess stomach bulge even after diet and exercise.

Pregnancy

Tummy tucks are usually an option for women after pregnancy and who do not plan to get pregnant again. A tummy tuck will not affect the pregnancy or the baby, according to the National Institutes of Health. Having a baby after a tummy tuck will affect the surgery results. The skin will stretch and lose muscle tone re□uiring another abdominoplasty to remove the excess skin to flatten the abdominal area. Therefore, this surgery is not recommended for women who are planning to get pregnant.

Side Effects of a Tummy Tuck

A tummy tuck, or abdominoplasty, is a major surgical procedure that involves removal of excess skin and fat, and restoration of weakened or separated muscles in the abdominal region. While a complete abdominoplasty is performed on those needing the most correction, a mini- or partial abdominoplasty may be performed on those needing shorter incisions whose fat deposits lie primarily under the naval.

Common side effects can vary in intensity and duration. Rarely, serious side effects can occur.

Common Side Effects

Individuals who have had a tummy tuck may experience some common side effects that can persist for a few weeks or even months. In the days following surgery, pain and swelling are likely to occur. Numbness and bruising are also common. These symptoms are sometimes severe enough to re□uire painkillers or other prescription medications. Patients are advised to avoid strenuous activity for six weeks or more to allow for proper healing, and this prolonged healing process can lead some to feel fatigued, emotionally drained or just otherwise not themselves.

Slow Healing and Scarring

Some patients may experience insufficient healing. Poor healing can lead to significant scarring, loss of skin or the need for a second surgery. Even among those who do heal normally, the scars caused by a tummy tuck may be prominent. In some cases, these scars will fade slightly over time, but they will never disappear. Certain topical creams may be prescribed by your surgeon to help reduce this scarring.

Bleeding and Infection

While a small amount of bleeding and leakage may normally occur around the wound site following a tummy tuck, bleeding under the skin flap can sometimes become severe, and re□uire prompt medical attention to prevent significant blood loss or other complications.

Infection is also possible, and if not treated promptly, the infection may spread throughout the body. Signs of an infection can include fever, chills, weakness, general malaise (feeling ill), and sweating. To help reduce the risk of infection, it is important to keep the wound clean by following the surgeon's instructions for cleaning the affected area regularly and changing its dressings. If infection is left untreated, the fatty tissue in the area of the wound may die (fatty necrosis), leading to skin loss and the possibility of spreading infection, according to the American Society of Plastic Surgeons.

Other Serious Side Effects

Though rare, serious side effects can occur as a result of undergoing surgery for a tummy tuck. Blood clots may develop in some people, and individuals who smoke or who have pre-existing health conditions such as diabetes or heart, lung or liver disease are at increased risk of developing blood clots. Blood clots that form and stay in a blood vessel can interfere with blood flow to various parts of the body. If the clot dislodges and travels to the brain, heart or lungs, it can lead to a stroke, heart attack or even death.

Reactions to the anesthesia

Some people can have severe reactions to anesthesia, particularly if they have never been placed under general anesthesia before. Any reaction will manifest itself immediately or within a day at the latest.

The American Society of Plastic Surgeons notes that other serious side effects that may occur include fluid accumulation in the extremities or abdomen, persistent swelling in the legs, nerve damage and aesthetic effects such as skin discoloration and prolonged swelling around the wound, recurrent looseness of skin, and asymmetries and unevenness of skin in the abdominal region.

Chapter 8

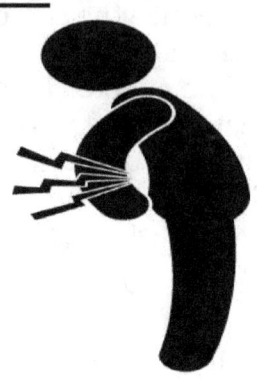

SIGNS YOU MIGHT NEED A TUMMY TUCK REVISION

Despite all the hard work involved to reach your ideal target weight, there are some things that diet and exercise won't affect, such as separated abdominal muscles or loose skin. As frustrating as this may be, at least abdominoplasty and other body contouring procedures offer a solution for these concerns.

But if your tummy tuck results don't live up to your expectations, what can you do? Here are three signs that you might be a good candidate for tummy tuck revision surgery.

1. You Notice Irregular Contours

Muscle laxity following pregnancy and loose skin left behind after significant weight loss are the two primary reasons men and women pursue tummy tucks. During surgery, your surgeon can repair and tighten those muscles, and then remove excess skin and tissue to reveal smoother, slimmer contours throughout the lower abdomen.

In some cases, though, your post-surgical silhouette may look uneven or may have too much fullness in the upper abdomen, typically due to an imbalance in skin tension after surgery. Choosing a highly skilled plastic surgeon with experience performing tummy tucks will minimize the chances of contour irregularity. Additionally, opting for a combination tummy tuck plus liposuction allows for more finesse during surgery, with the additional benefits of a drain-free tummy tuck.

2. Your Incision Looks Too High

When looking through before and after patient photos, you're likely to see incision placements ranging from below the bikini line to about halfway between the navel and pubic area. Regardless of how well an incision may heal up after recovery, a more discreet initial placement is definitely preferable for most patients.

The primary abdominoplasty incision should run from hip to hip across the lowest part of the belly where it will be fully hidden by everyday clothing. More ideally, the incision should be placed well enough that the scar is not visible even if wearing underwear or a swim suit... including a bikini. If you feel your incision is placed too high or you're unhappy with the appearance of your scar after healing, a tummy tuck revision may be able to help.

3. You're Unhappy with Your New Navel

A poorly re-created belly button can be one of the telltale signs of having had a tummy tuck. A too-shallow navel may look odd and obviously surgical, while a misshapen one is often the result of too much tension in the skin, which pulls and distorts the new belly button. Placement of the navel can appear either too high or too low on the belly as well.

Belly button revision (the technical term is umbilicoplasty) may be performed without the need for a secondary abdominoplasty. This relatively minor surgery can make a very positive aesthetic impact on the overall results of an otherwise satisfactory tummy tuck, or can also serve as the finishing touch in combination with a full tummy revision.

Choose the Right Surgeon

As important as it is to find a skilled and experienced plastic surgeon for your initial tummy tuck, it's even more critical for a revision surgery. Examine photos of prospective surgeons' work to ensure that the results reflect the natural contours of the abdomen rather than looking unnaturally flat, and take note of incision placement and how the belly button looks. With careful consideration and the right surgeon, you can enjoy beautiful, natural results even if it's the second time around.

Chapter 9

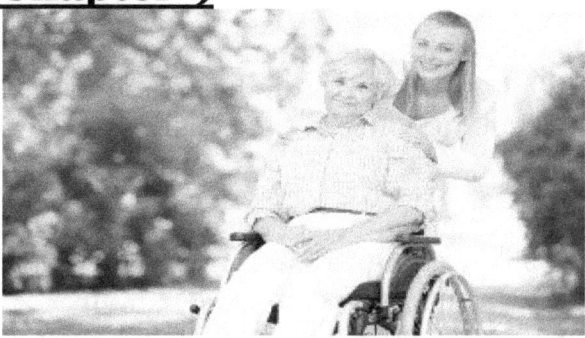

TUMMY TUCK RECOVERY

Tummy tuck or abdominoplasty surgery is a major surgical procedure. As with any major surgical procedure, recovery can take anything from a couple of weeks to a couple of months. You can generally expect for a year to pass before you can fully enjoy the benefits of a tummy tuck.

A tummy tuck aims to tighten the abdomen walls and muscles. It is also a procedure done to trim excess fat from the abdomen. The end result is often a nice trim abdomen with a manageable waistline.

Although some people think that a tummy tuck is a magical solution to help them lose a lot of weight, this simply isn't true. Tummy tucks are most effective on people with problems in the abdominal area and are within 30% of their calculated ideal body weight. A good surgeon will almost always refuse to perform a tummy tuck on an obese person. The risks are too great and the end result cannot be guaranteed.

Pregnancy is another big factor that will have an impact on a tummy tuck. Pregnancy puts a lot of pressure on the abdominal walls, which could undo a tummy tuck. Even after going through all planned pregnancies, the body needs time to recover. It is important to observe this recovery time to ensure that the abdomen is healthy and strong before enduring a major surgery.

Recovering from a tummy tuck is similar to recovering from any major surgery involving the abdomen. Give yourself a lot of time to fully heal before attempting to lift any heavy objects. Lifting heavy objects will put some stress on the abdominal muscles, and this could result in injury to the already scarred muscles.

Keep up a regular amount of fluid intake to ensure proper hydration. This is especially true immediately after surgery. The surgeon might limit your fluid intake in the beginning because a tummy tuck surgery is normally done under general anesthesia. However, your fluid intake is compensated with an IV drip.

Another important thing to take note is that you need to get out of bed as soon as you can and move about after your tummy tuck surgery. This movement will help to promote the healing of your wounds, and will speed up your recovery time by ensuring good blood circulation. Lying prone in bed after a major surgery is actually one of the worst things that you can do.

Chapter 10

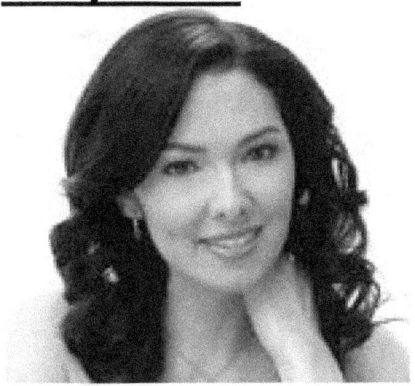

TUMMY TUCK QUESTIONS AND ANSWERS

This chapter provides answers to fre□uently asked abdominoplasty/ tummy tuck □uestions.

What is an abdominoplasty?

An abdominoplasty or tummy tuck is a surgical procedure that removes excess fat and skin from the abdomen and can also tighten your abdominal muscles. The result is a tighter looking abdominal area. Some patients re□uire repositioning of their belly button (umbilicus) through a new opening in the skin. The procedure can also remove or reduce the appearance of stretch marks and unwanted scars on your abdomen.

How do I know if I need an abdominoplasty?

You may be a candidate for an abdominoplasty if you are close to your ideal weight, but you still have excessive abdominal skin or bulging which you can't get rid of. This commonly results from having had multiple pregnancies or as a result of significant, often rapid weight loss. A decision to undergo an abdominoplasty procedure will ultimately have to made after careful consultation with your plastic surgeon.

Will a tummy tuck remove stretch marks?

Yes and no. If the stretch marks are in the lower abdomen (below the belly button), then a tummy tuck will get rid of them. However any stretch marks above the belly button will be pulled down onto the lower abdomen and may be stretched further. They can, however, end up looking smoother and flatter.

What are the different types of tummy tuck procedures?

Broadly speaking there are three types of tummy tuck procedure:

Standard

Mini

Extended

They all involve removing variable amounts of skin and fat (resulting in variable length scars), and all of them may or may not involve tightening of the abdominal muscles.

What is a standard abdominoplasty?

A standard or full abdominoplasty involves removing the excess skin and fat of the abdominal wall between the pubic area (bikini line in women), and the umbilicus. The umbilicus is left in its place, but a cut is made around it to free the surrounding skin. The remaining skin of the abdominal wall at the level of the umbilicus is then pulled down to suture it at the pubic level. The umbilicus is brought out through a new incision made in the skin that has been pulled down over it. The patient is left with a long, usually curved scar across the lower part of the abdominal wall at the level of the pubic hair. There is also a scar around the umbilicus. Any weakness of the abdominal muscles or hernias are repaired before the skin is closed.

What is a mini abdomioplasty?

A mini abdominoplasty is performed when there is minimal excess of skin and fat affecting the lower part of the abdomen. The excess skin and fat from below the umbilicus is removed; leaving a long curved scar on your abdomen just above the pubic area. The umbilicus remains undisturbed. Again, any laxity or hernia of the abdominal wall is repaired at the same time. The scar from a mini abdominoplasty is usually shorter than that of a standard abdominoplasty.

An apronectomy is a modification of the mini abdominoplasty for patients who have a large overhang of skin and fat over the pubic area. In this procedure only the surplus skin and fat is removed. The scar is long and extends from one side of the apron to the other.

What is an extended abdominoplasty?

Extended abdominoplasty is usually re□uired after massive weight loss. It involves removal of excess skin and fat from the abdomen and lower back. It will leave a scar around the umbilicus and a long curved scar on the abdomen above the pubic area, and around the lower back. Sometimes the scar extends the whole way around the body - circumferential abdominoplasty and this is a very major and involved procedure.

Is liposuction combined with abdominoplasty?

Liposuction is commonly combined with any of the different abdominoplasty procedures. Some surgeons prefer to perform liposuction at a later date.

Can I have liposuction alone instead of an abdominoplasty?

Sometimes liposuction alone can achieve a good result on the abdomen. A very important factor is the □uality of the patient's skin. Dramatic improvements can be achieved when the skin is of good □uality, and has not been overly stretched in the past. Skin □uality often determines whether liposuction alone will suffice or whether a combined surgical procedure will be needed.

What are the side effects of a tummy tuck?

As with all surgical procedures, there are risks associated with abdominoplasty surgery. Some patients are at higher risk of complications than others (for example smokers and patients who are over weight). You surgeon will be able to point out particular risks that you may be more susceptible to depending on your personal history and circumstances.

All patients will experience:

A variable degree of pain and bruising for at least a few days. Pain is usually worse if there has been a re□uirement to tighten your abdominal muscles (rectus plication).

A variable degree of swelling - this can take several months to completely subside.

Permanent scarring - the □uality of scarring cannot be guaranteed and usually depends on the way your body heals. Some patients can form thick, red, itchy scars, but most scarsusually fade over time (but won't completely disappear).

A variable degree of numbness of the skin over your abdomen - the skin below your new belly button may be numb for several months (if you have had a standard or extended abdominoplasty), but this numbness will gradually disappear as the nerves regrow.

What are the possible complications of a tummy tuck?

Complications can occur during or after the operation.

Possible general complications include an unexpected reaction to the anaesthetic, excessive bleeding or developing a blood clot, usually in a vein in the leg (deep vein thrombosis, DVT). A DVT can be a serious condition, and if the clot spreads to the lungs (pulmonary embolus) then the outcome can be fatal. Fortunately the incidence of pulmonary embolism after abdominoplasty is very rare (2 out of every 10,000 patients).

Complications specific to tummy tuck include:

Infection - this may need antibiotic treatment.

Bleeding (haematoma) - this may a return to theatre to stop the bleeding and drain the area.

Delayed wound healing - particularly in the tighter central part of the wound and sometimes dressings are needed for a few weeks. This is more common in patients who are overweight and who smoke.

Seroma - is a persistent collection of serous fluid under your skin after the drains have been removed. The fluid can be drained with a needle during your post-operative visits. Such drainage generally stops eventually (but may last for more than a month), and usually does not affect the final results. The incidence of seroma has been reported as affecting between 2-8 out of every 100 patients.

Poor scarring - scars can sometimes be red, thickened and itchy (hypertrophic scars). These can take several months to settle and fade.

Permanent numbness - numbness is usually temporary, but can be permanent.

Asymmetry - perfect symmetry does not exist before or after abdominoplasty surgery. Scars will never be identical from side to side, and the umbilicus will not be exactly in the midline.

Revisional surgery - secondary procedures are occasionally re☐uired to revise scars or to excise more skin (particularly on the sides).

How long does it take to recover from an abdominoplasty?

It usually takes about six weeks to make a full recovery from a tummy tuck, but this varies between individuals and the techni☐ue used. Over the counter pain killers such as paracetamol and ibuprofen are usually sufficient in the few days after your surgery. Patients can usually return to work about three to four weeks after their operation.

You will usually be able to do light activities at around 10 days after your surgery. Any vigorous activity should be avoided for at least six weeks. Your surgeon will give you specific instructions depending on the type of operation you have had.

What if I get pregnant after a tummy tuck?

Getting pregnant after a tummy tuck will not harm you or your baby, however it will undo (to some extent) the effects of your tummy tuck. If you are planning on getting pregnant it is best to wait until you have completed your family before undergoing a tummy tuck.

Chapter 11

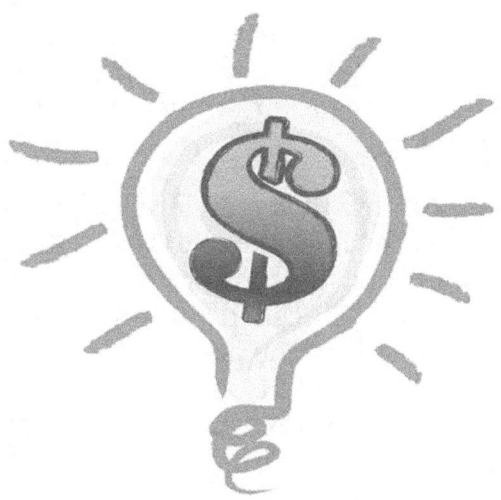

HOW MUCH DOES A TUMMY TUCK COST

A tummy tuck is a major surgical procedure that is performed to tighten and sculpt the abdominal region. The costs that are involved in a tummy tuck depend on several factors, some of which includes the age of the patient, the patient's body weight and the overall state of health. When budgeting for a tummy tuck surgery, it is also important to take into account all the costs that surround the procedure as well.

The best reference point when in□uiring about the costs that are involved in a tummy tuck surgery would be the surgeon himself. The surgeon will not only be able to explain all the procedures involved in the tummy tuck surgery, he will also be able to explain to you how your hard earned money will be spent in your tummy tuck. This will give you a better understanding of the costs involved.

When diagnosing you for a possible tummy tuck, the surgeon will able to determine if the tummy tuck procedure will be a simple one or a complex one. This will tie into the decision of possible medical prescriptions that could be involved. An anesthetist will also be involved in your tummy tuck. A simple tummy tuck can be done with local anesthetics while a complex one will be done under general anesthetics. All these factors will weigh in heavily in your final cost calculations. Even at the cheapest end of the scale, a tummy tuck will still run up to a few thousand dollars.

A lot of people who want a tummy tuck done are looking at overseas specialists because they have come to realize that the costs of a tummy tuck in places such as France or Italy is much less than the US or even the UK. So-called "tummy tuck holidays" are born from the needs of the people who not only want to find cheaper alternatives, but also from people who want to spend the recovery period away from home. Another reason would be to have a tummy tuck done away from prying eyes and nosey noses.

Conclusion

Thank you again for choosing this book!

A tummy tuck, also known as abdominoplasty, is a cosmetic surgery designed to remove excess skin and fat from the abdominal region that may accumulate due to the effects of pregnancy, obesity, or age.

 A tummy tuck also restores stretches or weakened abdominal muscles. Tummy tuck operations have been increasing in popularity and more and more men and women is having this procedure done.

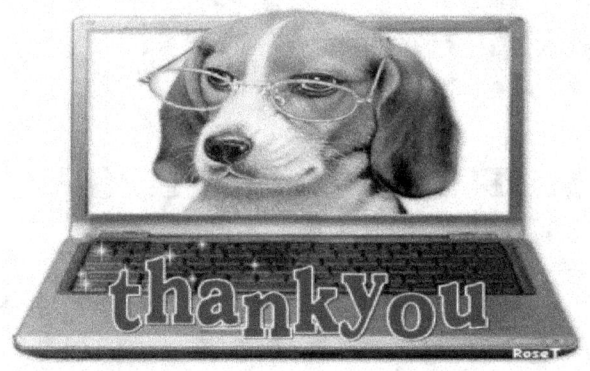

Finally, if you enjoyed this book, then I'd like to ask you for a favor, would you be kind enough to leave a review for this book on Amazon? It'd be greatly appreciated!

Thank you and good luck!

Preview Of 'COSMETIC SURGERY: WHAT YOU NEED TO DO BEFORE AND AFTER COSMETIC SURGERY'

Chapter 1

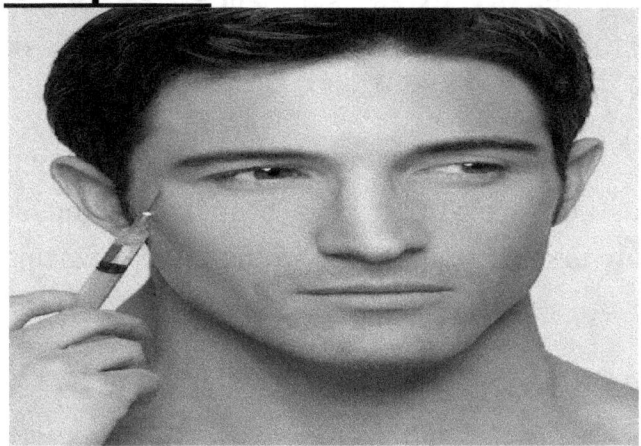

IS COSMETIC SURGERY A NEW PHENOMENON FOR MEN?

Cosmetic surgery isn't as new an idea as it may seem. It was first developed in India around 2000 BC. Surgery for aesthetic purposes crossed a major threshold in terms of popularity with the development of the Hollywood film industry; as today, many film actors and actresses achieved their "sculpted" features at least in part through cosmetic surgery.

Now, a wide variety of procedures are practiced around the world, and are priced in such a way that millions of people have been able to undergo cosmetic surgery in the last few years alone.

According to the American Society for Aesthetic Plastic Surgery, in the US alone, in the year 2008, over 17 million cosmetic surgical procedures were performed, and 90% of patients were women, but the proportion of men undergoing cosmetic surgery continues to increase yearly as well, which may be partly because corresponding stigmas have become less pronounced, and males are now expected to be concerned about their appearance as well.

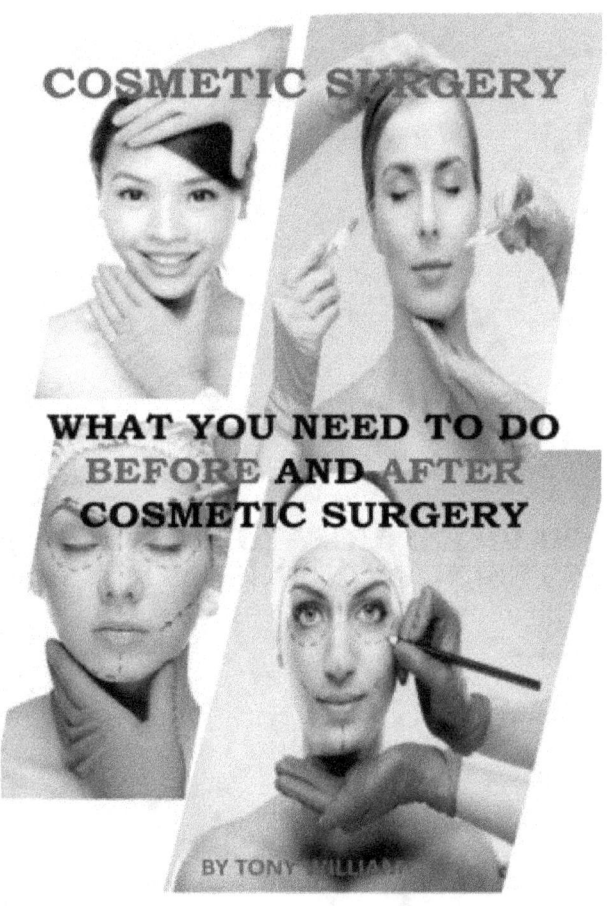

To check out the rest of (COSMETIC SURGERY: WHAT YOU NEED TO DO BEFORE AND AFTER COSMETIC SURGERY) go to Amazon.com

Check Out My Other Books

Below you'll find some of my other popular books that are popular on Amazon and Kindle as well. Alternatively, you can visit my author page on Amazon to see other work done by me.

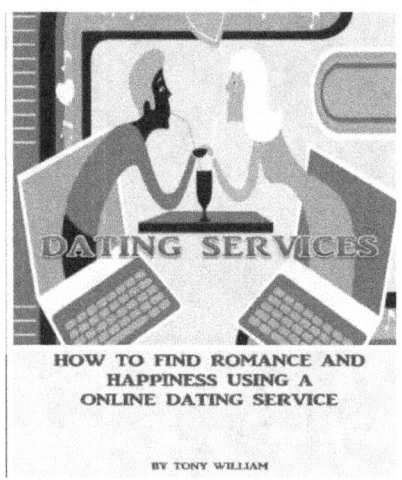

DATING SERVICES: HOW TO FIND ROMANCE AND HAPPINESS USING A ONLINE DATING SERVICE.

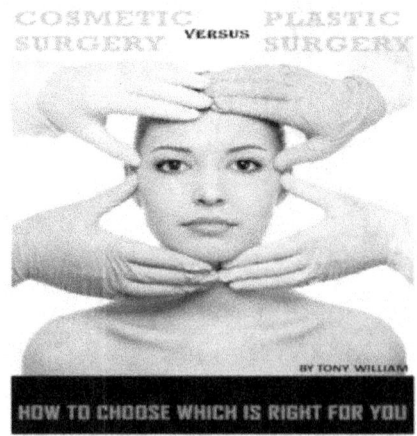

COSMETIC SURGERY VS. PLASTIC SURGERY: HOW TO CHOOSE WHICH IS RIGHT FOR YOU.

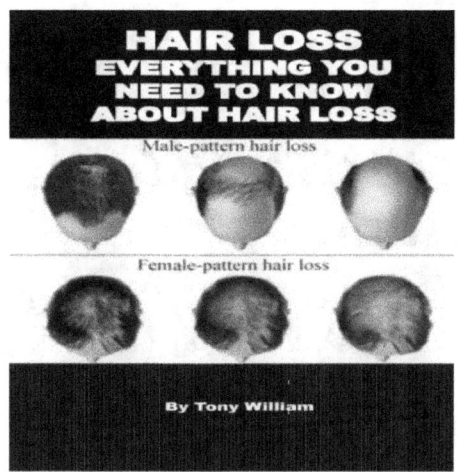

HAIR LOSS: EVERYTHING YOU NEED TO KNOW ABOUT HAIR LOSS.

BONUS: SUBSCRIBE TO THE FREE BOOK

Beginners Guide to Yoga & Meditation

"Stressed out? Do You Feel Like The World Is Crashing Down Around You? Want To Take A Vacation That Will Relax Your Mind, Body And Spirit? Well this Easy To Read Step By Step

E-Book Makes It All Possible!"

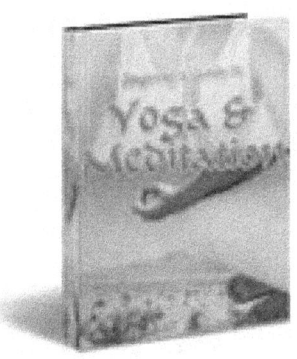

Instructions on how to join our mailing list, and receive a free copy of "Yoga and Meditation" can be found in any of my Kindle eBooks.

NOTES

NOTES

www.ingramcontent.com/pod-product-compliance
Lightning Source LLC
Chambersburg PA
CBHW071238220526
45468CB00002B/913